Nail Fungus

A Beginner's Quick Start Guide to Managing Nail Fungus Through Diet, With Sample Recipes and a 7-Day Meal Plan

mf

copyright © 2022 Patrick Marshwell

All rights reserved No part of this book may be reproduced, or stored in a retrieval system, or transmitted in any form or by any means, electronic, mechanical, photocopying, recording, or otherwise, without express written permission of the publisher.

Disclaimer

By reading this disclaimer, you are accepting the terms of the disclaimer in full. If you disagree with this disclaimer, please do not read the guide.

All of the content within this guide is provided for informational and educational purposes only, and should not be accepted as independent medical or other professional advice. The author is not a doctor, physician, nurse, mental health provider, or registered nutritionist/dietician. Therefore, using and reading this guide does not establish any form of a physician-patient relationship.

Always consult with a physician or another qualified health provider with any issues or questions you might have regarding any sort of medical condition. Do not ever disregard any qualified professional medical advice or delay seeking that advice because of anything you have read in this guide. The information in this guide is not intended to be any sort of medical advice and should not be used in lieu of any medical advice by a licensed and qualified medical professional.

The information in this guide has been compiled from a variety of known sources. However, the author cannot attest to or guarantee the accuracy of each source and thus should not be held liable for any errors or omissions.

You acknowledge that the publisher of this guide will not be held liable for any loss or damage of any kind incurred as a result of this guide or the reliance on any information provided within this guide. You acknowledge and agree that you assume all risk and responsibility for any action you undertake in response to the information in this guide.

Using this guide does not guarantee any particular result (e.g., weight loss or a cure). By reading this guide, you acknowledge that there are no guarantees to any specific outcome or results you can expect.

All product names, diet plans, or names used in this guide are for identification purposes only and are the property of their respective owners. The use of these names does not imply endorsement. All other trademarks cited herein are the property of their respective owners.

Where applicable, this guide is not intended to be a substitute for the original work of this diet plan and is, at most, a supplement to the original work for this diet plan and never a direct substitute. This guide is a personal expression of the facts of that diet plan.

Where applicable, persons shown in the cover images are stock photography models and the publisher has obtained the rights to use the images through license agreements with third-party stock image companies.

Table of Contents

Introduction — 7
What Is Nail Fungus? — 9
   Kinds of Nail Fungus — 10
Causes of Nail Fungus — 12
Symptoms of Nail Fungus — 14
How to Treat Nail Fungus Naturally — 16
   Treating Nail Fungus with Diet — 16
   Add More Protein, Fiber, and Quality Fats — 17
   Replenishing a Healthy Bacteria — 17
   Cutting the Root Cause: Yeast and Fungus — 18
   Takeaway — 20
   Topical Treatments — 20
   Other Methods — 22
   7-Day Meal Plan — 22
Sample Recipes — 24
   Apple and Onion Soup — 25
   Baked Tuna and Asparagus — 26
   Cinnamon and Orange Beef Stew — 27
   Shrimp Avocado Salad — 29
   Baked Spanish Mackerel Fillets — 31
   Miso Beef Noodle Soup — 32
   Pasta with Chard and White Bean — 34
   Kale, Lentils, and Onion Pasta — 36
   Avocado Egg Toast — 38
   Chia Seed and Strawberry Pudding — 39
   Anti-Diabetic Smoothie — 40
   Apple Cider Vinegar with Turmeric — 41
   Black Bean-Tomato Chili — 42
   Spinach and Chickpeas — 43

    Avocado and Caesar Salad   44
Prevention Tips for Nail Fungus   **45**
3-Step Plan for Managing Nail Fungus   **48**
    The Effectivity of Managing Nail Fungus through Natural Diet and Other Methods   49
Conclusion   **50**
FAQ   **51**
References and Helpful Links   **53**

Introduction

Nail Fungus is a common condition that can affect people of all ages. However, it is more common in seniors. This is because our nails become thicker and drier as we age, making them more susceptible to infection. Nail fungus can also be caused by certain medical conditions, such as diabetes or psoriasis.

This condition is not only unsightly, but it can also be painful. If left untreated, nail fungus can cause the nails to become brittle and even fall off.

If you have nail fungus, you may be self-conscious about the appearance of your nails. You may also be experiencing pain, redness, and swelling in the affected area. If left untreated, nail fungus can lead to serious health problems, such as cellulitis (skin infection) or paronychia (nail bed infection).

While there are many over-the-counter treatments for nail fungus, these can be expensive and may not work for everyone. Fortunately, there are some simple home remedies that can help treat nail fungus.

Luckily, there are several things seniors can do to clear up nail fungus and prevent it from coming back.

In this beginner's quick start guide, you will discover…

- What nail fungus is about
- Symptoms experienced in nail fungus
- How to prevent nail fungus
- Ways to treat nail fungus
- 3-step plan to manage nail fungus

What Is Nail Fungus?

Nail Fungus, also called Onychomycosis, is a common condition that affects toenails and fingernails. It is caused by a group of fungi called dermatophytes. These fungi thrive in warm, moist environments such as locker rooms, public showers, and swimming pools. The fungus can also be spread from person to person.

Nail fungus can cause the nails to become thick, yellow, or ragged. The nails may also break easily. In severe cases, the nail can separate from the nail bed. This can be painful and make walking difficult.

Onychomycosis or nail fungus is more common in older adults. This is because the nails thicken with age and become dry and brittle, making the nails more likely to crack easily. As soon as they do, fungi are able to enter the cracked nails easily. Also associated with age are slower blood circulation and a weakened immune system.

Another cause of Onychomycosis is athlete's foot. This is a fungal infection that affects the skin on the feet. It can spread to the nails if it is not treated. Athlete's foot is more common in men than women. Psoriasis is also another risk factor for nail fungus.

People with diabetes or a weakened immune system are more likely to develop serious complications from nail fungus. These complications can include cellulitis (skin infection) or paronychia (nail bed infection).

Nail fungus is not a serious health threat. However, it can be difficult to treat and can cause the nails to become discolored, thick, and brittle. If you have nail fungus, you may be self-conscious about the appearance of your nails. You may also be experiencing pain, redness, and swelling in the affected area.

If left untreated, nail fungus can lead to serious health problems, such as cellulitis (skin infection) or paronychia (nail bed infection).

If you have nail fungus, it is important to see a doctor. This is because the condition can be difficult to treat and can lead to other serious health problems.

Kinds of Nail Fungus

There are three main types of nail fungus:

Distal Subungual Onychomycosis (DSO)

This type of nail fungus is the most common. It affects the toenails more often than the fingernails. The fungus begins at the end of the nail and works its way under the nail. As the fungus grows, it causes the nail to become thick and discolored.

White superficial Onychomycosis (WSO)

This type of nail fungus affects the top layer of the nail. It is more common in fingernails than toenails. The nails may become white or yellow and have a powdery texture.

Proximal Subungual Onychomycosis (PSO)

This type of nail fungus begins at the base of the nail and works its way up. It is more common in toenails than fingernails. The nails may become thick, yellow, or ragged.

Nail fungus can be difficult to treat. This is because the nails are slow-growing, and the fungus can live deep within the nail. If you have nail fungus, it is important to see a doctor. They can prescribe medication to help clear up the infection. However, they can also be managed naturally through diet and other methods.

Causes of Nail Fungus

One of the causes of nail fungus is a weakened immune system. As you age, your immune system becomes weaker and is not able to protect your body as well as it used to. This makes you more susceptible to developing nail fungus. Another cause of nail fungus is poor circulation.

As you age, your circulation decreases, and this can lead to the development of nail fungus. Finally, another cause of nail fungus is trauma to the nails. This can happen if you injure your nails or if you frequently wear tight-fitting shoes that rub against your nails.

Another cause of Onychomycosis is Athlete's foot. This is a fungal infection that often affects the feet and can spread to the nails if it is not treated. Athletes' foot is often caused by moisture, so it is important to keep your feet dry. Wearing sandals or open-toed shoes can help prevent the spread of the Athlete's foot.

Common causes of nail fungus:

Nail fungus is often caused by a combination of factors, including sweating, poor hygiene, and trauma to the nail.

- *Sweating*: Sweating can contribute to nail fungus by providing a warm, moist environment for the fungus to grow.
- *Poor hygiene*: Poor hygiene habits can allow bacteria and fungi to thrive on the skin and nails.
- *Trauma to the nail*: Trauma to the nails, such as from nail-biting or manicures, can allow bacteria and fungi to enter the nails.
- *Athlete's foot*: Athlete's foot is a fungal infection that can spread to the nails if it is not treated.

Symptoms of Nail Fungus

Nail fungus, or onychomycosis, is a common nail disorder that affects seniors. The condition is caused by a fungal infection of the nails and can lead to pain, swelling, and discoloration of the nails. Nail fungus is often difficult to treat and can recur after treatment.

Symptoms of nail fungus include:

- Discoloration of the nails (yellow, brown, or white)
- Thickening of the nails
- Brittle or crumbly nails
- Foul odor coming from the nails
- Pain or discomfort in the affected area

Other symptoms include:

- Itchy skin around the nails
- Red, scaly skin around the nails
- Swollen skin around the nails

If you suspect that you have nail fungus, it is important to see a doctor or podiatrist for diagnosis and treatment. Nail fungus can be difficult to treat and may require oral antifungal medication, lasers, or other treatments. In some cases, nail fungus can lead to serious complications such as cellulitis or bone infections.

How to Treat Nail Fungus Naturally

As we age, our nails can become thicker and more brittle, making them more susceptible to fungus. While there are many commercial treatments available, they can be expensive and have potential side effects. Luckily, there are several natural ways to treat nail fungus.

Treating Nail Fungus with Diet

One of the best ways to fight nail fungus is through diet. Consuming foods that are high in antifungal properties can help to prevent and treat nail fungus. Because diet plays a role in overall immunity, it is also important to eat foods that support the immune system.

Also, be sure to drink plenty of fluids, as this will help to keep the nails hydrated and less susceptible to infection.

Some of the best antifungal foods include:

- garlic
- onions

- coconut oil
- apple cider vinegar
- ginger

Adding these foods to your diet can help keep fungus at bay.

Add More Protein, Fiber, and Quality Fats

Another way to fight nail fungus is by consuming more fiber, protein, and quality fats. These nutrients help to boost the immune system, which can help the body fight off fungal infections.

Some of the best sources of these nutrients include:

- beans
- nuts
- seeds
- avocados
- wild-caught fish
- grass-fed beef

Adding these foods to your diet can help improve your immune system and fight off nail fungus.

Replenishing a Healthy Bacteria

Another way to treat nail fungus is by replenishing healthy bacteria in the gut. This can be done by consuming probiotic-rich foods or taking a probiotic supplement.

Probiotics help to fight off bad bacteria and yeast, which can help to prevent and treat nail fungus.

Probiotics

Probiotics are live bacteria that are found in yogurt, fermented foods, and supplements. These bacteria can help to fight off infection and support the immune system. Some of the best sources of probiotics include:

- yogurt
- kefir
- sauerkraut
- kimchi
- miso soup
- tempeh

Taking a probiotic supplement is also a great way to get your daily dose of probiotics.

Cutting the Root Cause: Yeast and Fungus

One of the best ways to prevent and treat nail fungus is by cutting off the root cause, which is yeast and fungus. Eliminating what feeds the yeast because the candida virus lives in your digestive tract and among the common yeast grows, is the best way to prevent and treat nail fungus.

Yeast and fungus can be found in many different places, but they are most commonly found in the mouth, skin, and nails. People who have a weak immune system or suffer from diabetes are more susceptible to developing nail fungus. Nail fungus usually starts as a white or yellow spot on the tip of the nail. As the infection grows, the nail becomes discolored, thick, and brittle.

There are a few things you can do to cut off the root cause of nail fungus, which are yeast and fungus. One of the best ways to prevent and treat nail fungus is by eliminating what feeds the yeast and candida virus living in your digestive tract.

Some common foods that feed yeast are sugary foods, refined carbs, alcohol, and fermented foods. If you eliminate these foods from your diet, you will starve the yeast and Candida virus, which will help prevent and treat nail fungus.

Foods to avoid to prevent nail fungus:

- sugar
- bread
- alcohol
- dairy
- fried foods
- processed foods

You can also take supplements to help fight yeast and fungus. Some of the best supplements for this include:

- oregano oil
- berberine
- black walnut hulls

- goldenseal root
- tea tree oil
- caprylic acid

Takeaway

Nail fungus is a common condition that can cause pain, swelling, and discoloration of the nails. The condition is often difficult to treat and can recur after treatment.

There are several natural ways to treat nail fungus, including diet, supplements, and probiotics. Adding these foods and supplements to your diet can help to prevent and treat nail fungus.

Topical Treatments

In addition to dietary changes, several topical treatments can be effective in treating nail fungus. One of the most popular home remedies is tea tree oil. Tea tree oil has natural antifungal properties and can be applied directly to the affected nails.

Other essential oils that are effective against nail fungus include:

- peppermint oil
- oregano oil
- clove oil
- lavender oil

- Thyme oil

These oils can be diluted with a carrier oil and applied directly to the nails. Essential oils should not be taken orally.

Vinegar and water mixture

Soaking the nails in a mixture of vinegar and water can also help to kill fungus. Vinegar is a natural antiseptic and can help to prevent the growth of fungi.

For this treatment, mix one part vinegar with two parts of warm water and soak the nails for 15 minutes each day.

Snakeroot extract

Another option is to apply Snakeroot extract to the nails. This extract is effective against toenail fungus. It can be applied directly to the nails and allowed to dry.

Baking soda

This can also be used to treat nail fungus. It has antifungal and anti-inflammatory properties that can help to soothe the skin.

To use this remedy, mix one tablespoon of baking soda with two cups of warm water. Soak the nails in the mixture for 20 minutes each day.

Other Methods

In addition to diet and topical treatments, several other methods can be used to treat nail fungus. One of these is the following:

Increased air circulation around the nails.

Fungi thrive in moist, dark environments. By keeping the nails dry and exposing them to more air, you can create an environment that is less conducive to fungal growth.

Wearing socks and shoes that are made from breathable materials.

This can also help to prevent the growth of nail fungus. This is because fungi thrive in warm, damp environments. Wearing shoes and socks that allow air to circulate can help to keep the nails dry and reduce the chances of fungal growth.

If you have nail fungus, it is important to take action to treat it.

By making some simple dietary changes and using topical treatments, you can effectively manage nail fungus. If these methods do not work, there are several other options available to you. With diligence and perseverance, you can clear up your nail fungus and enjoy healthy, attractive nails.

7-Day Meal Plan

Here is a sample meal plan made for a week that you can either follow or modify accordingly. The meals listed below are lifted from the sample recipes included in this guide. The purpose of creating a meal plan is to help you to watch what you are about to consume and make sure you're meeting your daily nutrition needs.

	Breakfast	Lunch	Dinner
Day 1	Apple Cider Vinegar with Turmeric	Cinnamon and Orange Beef Stew	Avocado and Caesar Salad
Day 2	Avocado Egg Toast	Spinach and Chickpeas	Pasta with Chard and White Bean
Day 3	Anti-Diabetic Smoothie	Baked Tuna and Asparagus	Miso Beef Noodle Soup
Day 4	Chia Seed and Strawberry Pudding	Baked Spanish Mackerel Fillets	Black Bean-Tomato Chili
Day 5	Shrimp Avocado Salad	Kale, Lentils, and Onion Pasta	Apple and Onion Soup
Day 6	Avocado and Caesar Salad	Miso Beef Noodle Soup	Baked Tuna and Asparagus
Day 7	Avocado Egg Toast	Pasta with Chard and White Bean	Cinnamon and Orange Beef Stew

Sample Recipes

Apple and Onion Soup

Ingredients:

- 3 organic apples, diced
- 2 medium yellow onions, sliced
- 6 cups vegetable broth
- 1 small leek, chopped
- 1 tbsp. avocado oil
- 1/2 tbsp. fresh rosemary, chopped
- 1/2 tbsp. fresh thyme

Instructions:

1. Place the saucepan over medium heat.
2. Pour the avocado oil into the saucepan.
3. Add the onion slices. Sauté until the color has turned golden.
4. Pour in the vegetable broth.
5. Bring to a boil over medium heat.
6. Add the diced apples.
7. Reduce the heat to the medium-low setting.
8. Simmer for 10 minutes.
9. Serve immediately.

Baked Tuna and Asparagus

Ingredients:

- 2 5-oz. tuna fillets
- 14 oz. young potatoes
- 8 asparagus spears, trimmed and halved
- 2 handfuls of cherry tomatoes
- 1 handful fresh basil leaves
- 2 tbsp. extra-virgin olive oil
- 1 tbsp. balsamic vinegar

Instructions:

1. Heat oven to 428°F.
2. Arrange potatoes in a baking dish. Drizzle with a tablespoon of extra-virgin olive oil.
3. Roast potatoes for 20 minutes, or until golden brown.
4. Place the asparagus into the baking dish together with the potatoes. Roast in the oven for another 15 minutes.
5. Arrange the cherry tomatoes and tuna among the vegetables. Drizzle with balsamic vinegar and the remaining olive oil.
6. Roast for 10 to 15 minutes, or until tuna is cooked.
7. Throw in a handful of basil leaves before transferring everything to a serving dish. Serve while hot.

Cinnamon and Orange Beef Stew

Ingredients:

- 2 lbs. beef
- 3 cups beef broth
- 2 whole bay leaves
- 1 tsp. sage
- 1 tsp. rosemary
- 1 tsp. soy sauce
- 1 tsp. fish sauce
- 3 tbsp. coconut oil
- Orange zest
- 1 onion, chopped
- Orange juice
- 1 tsp. salt
- 1-1/2 tsp. black pepper
- 2 tsp. erythritol
- 2 tsp. ground cinnamon
- 2 tbsp. Apple cider vinegar
- 1 tbsp. fresh thyme
- 2-1/2 tsp. minced garlic

Instructions:

1. Cut vegetables into dice and the meat into cubes.
2. Heat the oil in a skillet and add meat. Do this in sets. Cook until brown.

3. After the last batch, add vegetables and cook for 2-3 minutes.
4. Deglaze the pan by adding orange juice.
5. Add all the remaining ingredients, except for the thyme, sage, and rosemary.
6. Cook for 1-2 minutes and transfer the mixture to a crockpot.
7. Cook on high for 2-3 hours.
8. Gently open the crockpot and add rosemary, sage, and thyme.
9. Cook for another 2 hours on high.
10. Serve while hot.

Shrimp Avocado Salad

Ingredients:

Salad:

- 1/2 lb. large shrimp, peeled
- 2 sweet corn ears, removed from the cob
- 4 cups Romaine lettuce, chopped
- 3 strips of bacon, diced
- 1 avocado, peeled, pitted and diced
- Optional: 1/3 cup Fontina cheese, grated

Buttermilk pesto dressing:

- 1/2 cup buttermilk
- 1/4 cup pesto, homemade or store-bought
- 1/2 cup mayo or Greek yogurt
- 1 tbsp. lemon juice
- 1 small shallot, minced
- salt
- pepper

Instructions:

1. Over high heat, place a skillet.
2. Put in the corn kernels when the skillet heats up.
3. Allow to dry-roast while stirring occasionally. Cook until the edges start to caramelize and turn brown about 6-8 minutes.
4. Place the roasted corn on a plate and set it aside.

5. Lower the heat to medium-high. Fry the bacon using the same skillet, for about 6 minutes, until crispy.
6. Transfer the bacon to a plate.
7. Saute the shrimp in the same skillet until they are cooked.
8. In a bowl, toss the lettuce, corn, avocado, bacon, and shrimp.
9. Whisk all the ingredients together until blended.
10. Season with salt and pepper.

Baked Spanish Mackerel Fillets

Ingredients:

- 6 pcs. Spanish mackerel filets
- 1/4 cup canola oil
- salt
- ground black pepper
- paprika
- 12 slices lemon

Instructions:

1. Arrange the oven rack so that it lies around 6 inches away from the source of heat.
2. Preheat the oven to 500°F.
3. Get a baking dish and lightly grease it.
4. Prepare each mackerel by rubbing both sides with canola oil.
5. Season the filets with salt, pepper, and paprika.
6. Top each filet with a couple of lemon slices.
7. Bake the filets for about 5 to 7 minutes, or just until the fish starts to flake.
8. Serve the fish right away.

Miso Beef Noodle Soup

Ingredients:

- 1/2 lb. flank steak, thinly sliced
- 2 carrots, peeled and thinly sliced
- 4 scallions, chopped
- 4 garlic cloves, minced
- 1/2 lb. shiitake mushrooms, stems removed and thinly sliced
- 1/4 cup cilantro, chopped
- 2 tbsp. mellow white miso paste
- 6 oz. udon or ramen noodles, cooked according to packaging instructions
- 2 cups of low-sodium beef broth
- 2 cups of packed baby spinach leaves
- 2 cups of water
- 1 tbsp. of canola oil

Instructions:

1. Place flank steak on a flat surface or plate.
2. Rub miso paste, garlic, and cilantro on both sides of the steak. Set aside.
3. Heat a large stockpot using the high setting. Add canola oil.
4. Place steak inside the pot.
5. Cook for 2 to 3 minutes or until the meat has turned brown on the outside.

6. Transfer the steak to a plate.
7. Add carrots, mushrooms, and scallions into the pot.
8. Cook while stirring often for 3 to 4 minutes or until mushrooms have begun to soften.
9. Add beef broth and water to the pot.
10. Reduce heat from high to low.
11. Add noodles and cover.
12. Cook while stirring occasionally for 2 to 3 minutes or until noodles are cooked through.
13. Add spinach.
14. Return the meat to the pot once the spinach leaves have wilted.
15. Transfer into serving bowls.
16. Serve immediately.

Pasta with Chard and White Bean

Ingredients:

- 1 can 15-1/2 oz. great northern beans, rinsed and drained
- 1 cup sweet onion, sliced
- 1 sweet potato, large, peeled and cut into 1/2" cubes
- 1 medium bunch Swiss chard, cut into 1" slices
- 1-12 oz. package penne pasta, whole wheat or brown rice
- 1 tbsp. balsamic vinegar
- 1 tbsp. fresh sage, minced or 1 tsp. sage, rubbed
- 1/3 cup fresh basil, chopped finely
- 1/4 tsp. chili powder
- 1/4 tsp. red pepper flakes, crushed
- 1/8 tsp. ground nutmeg
- 1/8 tsp. pepper
- 2 cups marinara sauce, warmed
- 2 tbsp. olive oil
- 3/4 tsp. salt
- 4 cups leeks, white portion only, sliced
- 4 garlic cloves, sliced

Instructions:

1. Cook pasta according to package directions.
2. Drain, reserving 3/4 cup pasta water.
3. In a stockpot, heat oil over medium heat.

4. Sauté leeks and onion until tender.
5. Add garlic and sage, cook and stir.
6. Add potato and chard.
7. Cover and cook over medium-low heat for about 5 minutes.
8. Stir in beans, dry seasonings, and reserved pasta water. Cover.
9. Leave to cook until chard and potato are tender.
10. Put in basil, pasta, and vinegar.
11. Toss well, allowing all the ingredients to heat through.
12. Serve with sauce.

Kale, Lentils, and Onion Pasta

Ingredients:

- 2-1/2 cups vegetable broth
- 3/4 cup dry lentils
- 1 tsp. salt
- 1 bay leaf
- 1/4 cup olive oil
- 1 large red onion, chopped
- 1 tsp. chopped fresh thyme
- 1/2 tsp. chopped fresh oregano
- 1/2 tsp. black pepper
- 1 bunch kale, stems removed and leaves coarsely chopped
- 1 pack of rotini pasta

Instructions:

1. In a saucepan, boil over high heat the following: vegetable broth, lentils, half teaspoon salt, and bay leaf.
2. Simmer down the heat to medium-low, cover, and then cook until the lentils are tender for about 20 minutes.
3. Add additional broth to keep the lentils moist if needed.
4. Discard the bay leaf once done.
5. As the lentils simmer, heat the olive oil in a skillet over medium-high heat.

6. Stir in the onion, thyme, oregano, pepper, and remaining salt. Stir-cook for a minute and add the sausage.
7. Reduce the heat to medium-low, and cook for 10 minutes.
8. Boil lightly salted water in a large pot over high heat.
9. Put in the kale and rotini pasta. Cook for 8 minutes until the rotini is firm.
10. Remove some of the cooking water, and set it aside.
11. Drain pasta then return to the pot.
12. Stir in the lentils and onion mixture.
13. Using the reserved cooking liquid, adjust the dish's moistness according to your preference.
14. Sprinkle with nutritional yeast to serve.

Avocado Egg Toast

Instructions:

- 1/4 avocado
- 1/8 tsp. garlic powder
- 1/4 tsp. ground pepper
- 1 pc. fried egg
- 1 slice toasted whole-wheat bread
- Optional: 1 tbsp. scallion
- Optional: 1 tsp. sriracha

Instructions:

1. Mash the avocado together with the garlic powder and pepper in a bowl.
2. Put the mashed avocado on the toast.
3. Add the egg on top then garnish with scallion and sriracha.
4. Serve immediately.

Chia Seed and Strawberry Pudding

Ingredients:

- 1 cup strawberries, thinly sliced
- 3 tbsp. chia seeds
- 1 cup soy beverage, unsweetened and fortified

Instructions:

1. To create pudding, combine the soy beverage and chia seeds.
2. Refrigerate the mixture for half an hour.
3. Stir the mixture every 5 minutes to prevent the chia seeds from sticking together.
4. As an alternative, blend the soy beverage and chia seeds in a food processor and let it chill in the refrigerator.
5. Slice strawberries lengthwise.
6. Pour chilled pudding into 2 glasses. Place the strawberry slices on top.
7. Serve and enjoy your pudding.

Anti-Diabetic Smoothie

Ingredients:

- 2 cups spinach
- 2 large kale leaves
- 3/4 cup water
- 1 large frozen banana
- 1/2 cup frozen mango
- 1/2 cup frozen peach
- 1 tablespoon ground flaxseeds
- 1 tablespoon almond butter or peanut butter

Instructions:

1. Using a blender, mix the water, spinach, and kale. Increase speed until all solid particles are gone.
2. Add the rest of the ingredients. Resume blending until reaching the maximum speed.
3. Maintain the maximum speed for 30 seconds before serving.
4. Serve chilled.

Apple Cider Vinegar with Turmeric

Ingredients:

- 1 tbsp. apple cider vinegar
- 1 tbsp. lemon juice, freshly squeezed
- 1/4 tsp. turmeric
- 1 cup hot or warm water
- 1/2 tbsp. pure maple syrup or honey

Instructions:

Mix all the ingredients and enjoy while warm.

Black Bean-Tomato Chili

Ingredients:

- 1 cup orange juice or juice from 3 medium oranges
- 1 onion, chopped
- 1 green pepper, chopped
- 1 tsp. chili powder
- 1 tsp. ground cinnamon
- 1 tsp. ground cumin
- 1/4 tsp. pepper
- 2 cans 15 oz. black beans, rinsed and drained
- 2 tbsp. olive oil
- 3 cans 14-1/2 oz. diced tomatoes, undrained
- 3 garlic cloves, minced

Instructions:

1. Heat oil over medium-high heat in a Dutch oven.
2. Saute green pepper and onion until tender, around 8 to 10 minutes.
3. Add in seasonings and garlic. Cook for a minute longer.
4. Stir in the remaining ingredients and bring to a boil.
5. Reduce heat. Allow to simmer while covered for 20-25 minutes. Stir occasionally.
6. Serve and enjoy while hot.

Spinach and Chickpeas

Ingredients:

- 3 tbsp. extra virgin olive oil
- 1 onion, thinly sliced
- 4 cloves garlic, minced
- 1 tbsp. grated ginger
- 1/2 container grape tomatoes
- 1 lemon, zested and freshly juiced
- 1 tsp. crushed red pepper flakes
- 1 large can of chickpeas
- 6 cups spinach
- Sea salt to taste

Instructions:

1. Add extra virgin olive oil to a large skillet, add onion, and cook until the onion starts to brown.
2. Add ginger, garlic, tomatoes, spinach, red pepper flakes, and lemon zest.
3. Allow to cook for about 3 to 4 minutes.
4. Add cooked chickpeas and stir. Add oil if necessary.
5. Serve and enjoy.

Avocado and Caesar Salad

Ingredients:

- 1 head romaine hearts, washed
- 1 package of tempeh
- 1 small red onion, chopped
- 1/2 avocado, sliced
- sea salt
- umeboshi vinegar

Instruction:

1. Place red onions in a bowl.
2. Add a dash of sea salt and about 3 drops of umeboshi vinegar.
3. Rub the salt and vinegar mixture very gently into the onion. Do so until the color deepens. Set aside.
4. Tear apart the lettuce and place it into a bowl.
5. Add in the red onion mixture, followed by the tempeh.
6. Toss the salad lightly using a wooden spoon or with your hands.
7. Add the avocado. Toss again.
8. Drizzle a dash of umeboshi vinegar over the salad. Toss to blend the ingredients.

Prevention Tips for Nail Fungus

Preventing nail fungus can be difficult, especially if you already have the condition. However, there are some things you can do to reduce your risk of developing nail fungus or of re-infecting yourself if you've already had the condition.

- Keep your nails clean and trimmed. This will help to prevent dirt and bacteria from getting under your nails and causing an infection.
- Avoid sharing nail clippers or other personal items with others. This is especially important if you know someone who has nail fungus.
- Wear socks and shoes that are made from breathable materials. This will help to keep your feet dry and reduce the risk of developing an athlete's foot, which can lead to nail fungus.
- Don't walk barefoot in public places. This includes showers, locker rooms, and pool areas. Walking barefoot puts you at risk of coming into contact with the fungus that causes nail fungus.

- Keep your feet dry as much as possible. This is especially important if you sweat a lot or have diabetes.
- Consider using an antifungal powder in your shoes. This can help to prevent the growth of fungus and keep your feet dry.
- Wear sandals or open-toed shoes when possible. This will help to keep your nails exposed to air and reduce the risk of developing nail fungus.
- Avoid using artificial nails. Artificial nails can provide a place for the fungus to grow and can be difficult to clean properly.
- If you get a pedicure, make sure the salon uses sterilized tools. This will help to prevent the spread of nail fungus.

Talk to your doctor about taking antifungal medication if you have a high risk of developing nail fungus. This is especially important if you have diabetes or a weakened immune system.

Taking these steps can help to prevent nail fungus or re-infection if you've already had the condition. However, it's important to see your doctor if you think you may have nail fungus so that it can be properly diagnosed and treated.

If you have nail fungus, there are some things you can do to help prevent the condition from worsening or coming back. These include:

- Wearing shoes that fit well and are made of breathable materials
- Keeping your feet clean and dry
- Avoiding moist environments (such as public showers)
- Wearing socks made of natural fibers
- Changing your socks frequently
- Not sharing nail clippers or other personal items
- Disinfecting any personal items that come into contact with your nails

3-Step Plan for Managing Nail Fungus

Now that you know what nail fungus is and what causes it let's get into how you can manage it. Here is a 3-step plan for managing your nail fungus:

1. Change your diet: The first step in managing your nail fungus is to change your diet. Eliminate sugary and processed foods from your diet and replace them with whole, nutritious foods. Consume plenty of fresh fruits and vegetables, as well as lean protein sources such as fish, chicken, tofu, and beans. Adding probiotic-rich foods to your diet can also be helpful in managing nail fungus.
2. Implement natural treatments: There are a number of natural treatments that can be effective in treating nail fungus. Some of these include tea tree oil, garlic, and oregano oil. You can also try soaking your feet in vinegar or Epsom salt baths.
3. See a doctor: If you have tried natural treatments and your nail fungus is still not improving, it is important

to see a doctor. A doctor can prescribe oral antifungal medication that is effective in treating nail fungus.

The Effectivity of Managing Nail Fungus through Natural Diet and Other Methods

Nail fungus is one of the most common problems that can affect both toenails and fingernails. It is caused by a group of fungi called dermatophytes which live on the dead tissues of the nails, skin, and hair. The condition is also known as onychomycosis or tinea unguium.

Nail fungus usually starts as a white or yellow spot on the tip of the nail. As the infection progresses, it may cause the nail to become thick, discolored, and brittle. The affected nails may also emit a foul odor. In severe cases, the nail may separate from the bed, which can be extremely painful.

Nail fungus is a very common condition that affects about 3% of the population. It is more common in adults but can also affect children. The condition is more prevalent in toenails than fingernails and is more common in men than women.

Conclusion

Nail fungus is a common problem, especially for seniors. However, it is important to remember that nail fungus is treatable. By following the steps outlined in this article, you can effectively manage your nail fungus and improve the appearance of your nails.

If you suspect that you have nail fungus, it is important to see a doctor or podiatrist for diagnosis and treatment. Nail fungus can be difficult to treat and may require oral antifungal medication, lasers, or other treatments. In some cases, nail fungus can lead to serious complications, so it is important to seek treatment as soon as possible.

FAQ

1. How common is nail fungus?

Nail fungus is very common, affecting about 3% of the population. It is more common in adults but can also affect children. The condition is more prevalent in toenails than fingernails and is more common in men than women.

2. What are the symptoms of nail fungus?

The symptoms of nail fungus include a white or yellow spot on the nail, thickening of the nail, discoloration of the nail, brittle nails, and foul-smelling nails. In severe cases, the nail may separate from the bed, which can be extremely painful.

3. What causes nail fungus?

Nail fungus is caused by a group of fungi called dermatophytes, which live on the dead tissues of the nails, skin, and hair.

4. How is nail fungus treated?

There are a number of treatments for nail fungus, including oral antifungal medication, lasers, and other treatments. In some cases, nail fungus can be difficult to treat and may require multiple treatments.

References and Helpful Links

"10 Home Remedies for Toenail Fungus." Healthline, 17 Feb. 2021, https://www.healthline.com/health/home-remedies-for-toenail-fungus. Accessed 15 July 2022.

Lose 10 Pounds in a Week? Is It Possible or Safe? 13 Apr. 2018, https://www.medicalnewstoday.com/articles/321493. Accessed 15 July 2022.

Nail Fungus: Diagnosis and Treatment. https://www.aad.org/public/diseases/a-z/nail-fungus-treatment. Accessed 15 July 2022.

"Nail Fungus - Symptoms and Causes." Mayo Clinic, https://www.mayoclinic.org/diseases-conditions/nail-fungus/symptoms-causes/syc-20353294. Accessed 15 July 2022.

"Skin Problems and Treatments." WebMD, https://www.webmd.com/skin-problems-and-treatments/default.htm. Accessed 15 July 2022.

"The 7 Best Toenail Fungus Treatments of 2022." Verywell Health, https://www.verywellhealth.com/best-toenail-fungus-treatments-4174023. Accessed 15 July 2022.

"Treating Toenail Fungus." EverydayHealth.Com, https://www.everydayhealth.com/hs/toenail-fungal-infection-guide/treating-toenail-fungus/. Accessed 15 July 2022.

"Toenail Fungus (Onychomycosis): Causes & Symptoms." Cleveland Clinic, https://my.clevelandclinic.org/health/diseases/11303-toenail-fungus. Accessed 15 July 2022.

www.ingramcontent.com/pod-product-compliance
Lightning Source LLC
LaVergne TN
LVHW051924060526
838201LV00062B/4673